Tomorrow's Doctors

Published September 2009

General
Medical
Council

Regulating doctors
Ensuring good medical practice

Contents

Foreword

Doctors must be capable of regularly taking responsibility for difficult decisions in situations of clinical complexity and uncertainty.

See Appendix 3, *Related documents*: 56

Medical schools equip medical students with the scientific background and technical skills they need for practice. But, just as importantly, they must enable new graduates to both understand and commit to high personal and professional values. Medicine involves personal interaction with people, as well as the application of science and technical skills.

In *Good Medical Practice* the GMC states:
'Good doctors make the care of their patients their first concern: they are competent, keep their knowledge and skills up to date, establish and maintain good relationships with patients and colleagues, are honest and trustworthy, and act with integrity.'

See GMC, *Good Medical Practice*, paragraph 1

Putting patients first involves working with them as partners in their own care and making their safety paramount. It involves dedication to continuing improvement, both in the doctor's individual practice and in the organisation and environment in which they work.

It is not enough for a clinician to act as a practitioner in their own discipline. They must act as partners to their colleagues, accepting shared accountability for the service provided to patients. They are also expected to offer leadership, and to work with others to change systems when it is necessary for the benefit of patients.[1]

In *Tomorrow's Doctors*, we cover these themes under three headings, relating to the doctor as a scientist and a scholar, as a practitioner, and as a professional. These categories cover the development of the knowledge, skills and behaviour students must demonstrate by the time they graduate. However, the categories and the specific outcomes should not be considered in isolation from each other. Doctors need to link them routinely in clinical practice.

Graduation is an early threshold in doctors' careers. New graduates cannot be expected to have the clinical experience, specialist expertise or leadership skills of a consultant or GP. But they must be able to demonstrate all the outcomes in *Tomorrow's Doctors* in order to be properly prepared for clinical practice and the Foundation Programme. The Foundation Programme builds on undergraduate education, allowing new doctors to demonstrate performance in the workplace. It includes a range of clinical experience which often involves caring for acutely ill patients.

See Appendix 3, *Related documents*: 32

The outcomes set out what the GMC expects medical schools to deliver and what the employers of new graduates can expect to receive although medical schools are free to require their graduates to demonstrate additional competences. These outcomes mark the end of the first stage of a continuum of medical learning that runs from the first day at medical school and continues until the doctor's retirement from clinical practice.

Professional regulation has changed dramatically since the first edition of *Tomorrow's Doctors* was published in 1993. The GMC has published *Good Medical Practice* and other guidance which sets out the positive standards expected of good doctors in the new world of partnership with patients and colleagues. Registration and fitness to practise procedures have been transformed. Licensing and revalidation will also support regulation, professional values and lifelong learning.

See GMC, *Good Medical Practice*

For this edition, among a number of important changes, we have responded specifically to concerns about scientific education, clinical skills, partnership with patients and colleagues, and commitment to improving healthcare and providing leadership. We have also set out standards for the delivery of medical education with a new emphasis on equality and diversity, involving employers and patients, the professional development of teaching staff, and ensuring that students derive maximum benefit from their clinical placements.

We realise that meeting these outcomes and standards will be challenging. There are implications for resources and priorities both for medical schools and for the health service. But the benefit will be a further enhancement of the knowledge, skills and behaviour which new graduates will bring to their practice.

Today's undergraduates – tomorrow's doctors – will see huge changes in medical practice. There will be continuing developments in biomedical sciences and clinical practice, new health priorities, rising expectations among patients and the public, and changing societal attitudes. Basic knowledge and skills, while fundamentally important, will not be enough on their own. Medical students must be inspired to learn about medicine in all its aspects so as to serve patients and become the doctors of the future. With that perspective and commitment, allied to the specific knowledge, skills and behaviours set out in *Tomorrow's Doctors* and *Good Medical Practice*, they will be well placed to provide and to improve the health and care of patients, as scholars and scientists, practitioners and professionals.

Professor Peter Rubin
Chair – General Medical Council

See GMC, *Good Medical Practice*

Introduction

1   The GMC, the medical schools, the NHS, doctors and students all have different and complementary roles in medical education.

2   The GMC is responsible for:

(a) Protecting, promoting and maintaining the health and safety of the public.

(b) Promoting high standards of medical education.

(c) Deciding on the knowledge, skills and behaviours required of graduates.

(d) Setting the standard of expertise that students need to achieve at qualifying examinations or assessments.

(e) Making sure that:

   i. the teaching and learning opportunities provided allow students to meet our requirements

   ii. the standard of expertise we have set is maintained by medical schools at qualifying examinations.

(f) Appointing inspectors of qualifying examinations and assessments to report on the standard of examinations and assessments, and on the quality of teaching and learning.

(g) Appointing visitors to medical schools and proposed medical schools, to report on the quality of teaching and learning.

(h) Recognising, continuing to recognise or no longer recognising individual UK Primary Medical Qualifications (PMQs), in the light of the outcome of quality assurance activities.

(i) Maintaining a list of bodies that, having satisfactorily demonstrated that they meet our requirements, are entitled to award PMQs.

(j) Removing bodies which have failed to meet our requirements from the list of those that are entitled to award PMQs.

(k) Considering applications under Section 10A(2)(f) of the Medical Act 1983 for arrangements for a person with a disability not to be disadvantaged unfairly by the disability when participating in a programme for provisionally registered doctors.

(l) From the introduction of the licence to practise, granting graduates provisional registration with a licence to practise, subject to their fitness to practise not being impaired.

3   Medical schools are responsible for:

(a)   Protecting patients and taking appropriate steps to minimise any risk of harm to anyone as a result of the training of their medical students.

(b)   Managing and enhancing the quality of their medical education programmes.

(c)   Delivering medical education in accordance with principles of equality.

(d)   Selecting students for admission.

(e)   Providing a curriculum and associated assessments that meet:

   i.   the standards and outcomes in *Tomorrow's Doctors*

   ii.   the requirements of the EU Medical Directive.

(f)   Providing academic and general support to students.

(g)   Providing support and training to people who teach and supervise students.

(h)   Providing appropriate student fitness to practise arrangements.

(i)   Ensuring that only students who demonstrate the outcomes set out in *Tomorrow's Doctors* are permitted to graduate.

(j)   Managing the curriculum and ensuring that appropriate education facilities are provided in the medical school and by other education providers.[2]

4   NHS organisations[3] are responsible for:

(a) Making available the facilities, staff and practical support needed to deliver the clinical parts of the curriculum.

(b) Ensuring that performance of teaching responsibilities is subject to appraisal.

(c) Including, when appropriate, a contractual requirement for doctors to carry out teaching.

(d) Releasing doctors and other staff to complete the training needed to be teachers, and to take part in professional development and quality assurance activities.

(e) Taking part in the management and development of the clinical education they carry out.

(f) Supporting medical schools in complying with *Tomorrow's Doctors*.

(g) Providing quality-control information to the medical school about their education provision.

5   Doctors are responsible for:

(a) Following the principles of professional practice that are set out in *Good Medical Practice*, including being willing to contribute to the education of students.

5a. See GMC, *Good Medical Practice*

(b) Developing the skills and practices of a competent teacher if they are involved in teaching.

5b. See GMC, *Good Medical Practice*, paragraphs 15-19; Appendix 3, *Related documents*: 39

(c) Supervising the students for whom they are responsible, to support their learning and ensure patient safety.

(d) Providing objective, honest and timely assessments of the students they are asked to appraise or assess.

(e) Providing feedback on students' performance.

(f) Meeting contractual requirements, including any that relate to teaching.

6 Students are responsible for:

(a) Their own learning, including achieving all the outcomes set out in *Tomorrow's Doctors*, whatever their personal preferences or religious beliefs.

(b) Ensuring patient safety by working within the limits of their competence, training and status as medical students.

(c) Raising any concerns about patient safety, or any aspect of the conduct of others which is inconsistent with good professional practice.

(d) Providing evaluations of their education for quality management purposes.

(e) Keeping to the guidance *Medical students: professional values and fitness to practise* developed by the GMC and the Medical Schools Council.

6c. See GMC, *Good Medical Practice*, paragraphs 6, 43-45; GMC, *Raising concerns about patient safety*

6e. See GMC and Medical Schools Council, *Medical students: professional values and fitness to practise*

Outcomes for graduates

Overarching outcome for graduates

7 Medical students are tomorrow's doctors. In accordance with *Good Medical Practice*, graduates will make the care of patients their first concern, applying their knowledge and skills in a competent and ethical manner and using their ability to provide leadership and to analyse complex and uncertain situations.

7. See GMC, *Good Medical Practice*, 'Duties of a Doctor' (also inside front cover of *Tomorrow's Doctors*)

Outcomes 1 – The doctor as a scholar and a scientist

8 The graduate will be able to apply to medical practice biomedical scientific principles, method and knowledge relating to: anatomy, biochemistry, cell biology, genetics, immunology, microbiology, molecular biology, nutrition, pathology, pharmacology and physiology. The graduate will be able to:

8. See Appendix 3, *Related documents:* 1, 2, 3, 8, 11

(a) Explain normal human structure and functions.

(b) Explain the scientific bases for common disease presentations.

(c) Justify the selection of appropriate investigations for common clinical cases.

(d) Explain the fundamental principles underlying such investigative techniques.

(e) Select appropriate forms of management for common diseases, and ways of preventing common diseases, and explain their modes of action and their risks from first principles.

(f) Demonstrate knowledge of drug actions: therapeutics and pharmacokinetics; drug side effects and interactions, including for multiple treatments, long-term conditions and non-prescribed medication; and also including effects on the population, such as the spread of antibiotic resistance.

8f. See Appendix 3, *Related documents*: 9, 10

(g) Make accurate observations of clinical phenomena and appropriate critical analysis of clinical data.

9 Apply psychological principles, method and knowledge to medical practice.

9. See Appendix 3, *Related documents*: 4, 12

(a) Explain normal human behaviour at an individual level.

(b) Discuss psychological concepts of health, illness and disease.

(c) Apply theoretical frameworks of psychology to explain the varied responses of individuals, groups and societies to disease.

(d) Explain psychological factors that contribute to illness, the course of the disease and the success of treatment.

(e) Discuss psychological aspects of behavioural change and treatment compliance.

(f) Discuss adaptation to major life changes, such as bereavement; comparing and contrasting the abnormal adjustments that might occur in these situations.

(g) Identify appropriate strategies for managing patients with dependence issues and other demonstrations of self-harm.

9g. See Appendix 3, *Related documents*: 7

10 Apply social science principles, method and knowledge to medical practice.

(a) Explain normal human behaviour at a societal level.
(b) Discuss sociological concepts of health, illness and disease.
(c) Apply theoretical frameworks of sociology to explain the varied responses of individuals, groups and societies to disease.
(d) Explain sociological factors that contribute to illness, the course of the disease and the success of treatment – including issues relating to health inequalities, the links between occupation and health and the effects of poverty and affluence.
(e) Discuss sociological aspects of behavioural change and treatment compliance.

11 Apply to medical practice the principles, method and knowledge of population health and the improvement of health and healthcare.

11. See Appendix 3, *Related documents*: 5, 57

(a) Discuss basic principles of health improvement, including the wider determinants of health, health inequalities, health risks and disease surveillance.

11a. See Appendix 3, *Related documents*: 37, 38

(b) Assess how health behaviours and outcomes are affected by the diversity of the patient population.

(c) Describe measurement methods relevant to the improvement of clinical effectiveness and care.

(d) Discuss the principles underlying the development of health and health service policy, including issues relating to health economics and equity, and clinical guidelines.

(e) Explain and apply the basic principles of communicable disease control in hospital and community settings.

(f) Evaluate and apply epidemiological data in managing healthcare for the individual and the community.

(g) Recognise the role of environmental and occupational hazards in ill-health and discuss ways to mitigate their effects.

(h) Discuss the role of nutrition in health.

(i) Discuss the principles and application of primary, secondary and tertiary prevention of disease.[4]

(j) Discuss from a global perspective the determinants of health and disease and variations in healthcare delivery and medical practice.

12   Apply scientific method and approaches to medical research.

12. See GMC, *Research*

(a)   Critically appraise the results of relevant diagnostic, prognostic and treatment trials and other qualitative and quantitative studies as reported in the medical and scientific literature.

(b)   Formulate simple relevant research questions in biomedical science, psychosocial science or population science, and design appropriate studies or experiments to address the questions.

(c)   Apply findings from the literature to answer questions raised by specific clinical problems.

(d)   Understand the ethical and governance issues involved in medical research.

Outcomes 2 – The doctor as a practitioner

13   The graduate will be able to carry out a consultation with a patient:

13. See Appendix 3, *Related documents*: 6

(a)   Take and record a patient's medical history, including family and social history, talking to relatives or other carers where appropriate.

(b)   Elicit patients' questions, their understanding of their condition and treatment options, and their views, concerns, values and preferences.

(c)   Perform a full physical examination.

(d)   Perform a mental-state examination.

(e)   Assess a patient's capacity to make a particular decision in accordance with legal requirements and the GMC's guidance.

13e. See GMC, *Consent: patients and doctors making decision together*, paragraphs 71-74

(f)   Determine the extent to which patients want to be involved in decision-making about their care and treatment.

(g)   Provide explanation, advice, reassurance and support.

14 Diagnose and manage clinical presentations.

(a) Interpret findings from the history, physical examination and mental-state examination, appreciating the importance of clinical, psychological, spiritual, religious, social and cultural factors.

(b) Make an initial assessment of a patient's problems and a differential diagnosis. Understand the processes by which doctors make and test a differential diagnosis.

(c) Formulate a plan of investigation in partnership with the patient, obtaining informed consent as an essential part of this process.

(d) Interpret the results of investigations, including growth charts, x-rays and the results of the diagnostic procedures in Appendix 1.

(e) Synthesise a full assessment of the patient's problems and define the likely diagnosis or diagnoses.

(f) Make clinical judgements and decisions, based on the available evidence, in conjunction with colleagues and as appropriate for the graduate's level of training and experience. This may include situations of uncertainty.

(g) Formulate a plan for treatment, management and discharge, according to established principles and best evidence, in partnership with the patient, their carers, and other health professionals as appropriate. Respond to patients' concerns and preferences, obtain informed consent, and respect the rights of patients to reach decisions with their doctor about their treatment and care and to refuse or limit treatment.

(h) Support patients in caring for themselves.

(i) Identify the signs that suggest children or other vulnerable people may be suffering from abuse or neglect and know what action to take to safeguard their welfare.

(j) Contribute to the care of patients and their families at the end of life, including management of symptoms, practical issues of law and certification, and effective communication and teamworking.

14j. See GMC, *Withholding and withdrawing life prolonging treatments*

15 Communicate effectively with patients and colleagues in a medical context.

15. See GMC, *Good Medical Practice*, paragraphs 22, 23, 27, 29, 41; Appendix 3, *Related documents*: 6, 24, 36, 40, 41

(a) Communicate clearly, sensitively and effectively with patients, their relatives or other carers, and colleagues from the medical and other professions, by listening, sharing and responding.

(b) Communicate clearly, sensitively and effectively with individuals and groups regardless of their age, social, cultural or ethnic backgrounds or their disabilities, including when English is not the patient's first language.

(c) Communicate by spoken, written and electronic methods (including medical records), and be aware of other methods of communication used by patients. The graduate should appreciate the significance of non-verbal communication in the medical consultation.

(d) Communicate appropriately in difficult circumstances, such as when breaking bad news, and when discussing sensitive issues, such as alcohol consumption, smoking or obesity.

(e) Communicate appropriately with difficult or violent patients.

(f) Communicate appropriately with people with mental illness.

(g) Communicate appropriately with vulnerable patients.

(h) Communicate effectively in various roles, for example, as patient advocate, teacher, manager or improvement leader.

16 Provide immediate care in medical emergencies.

(a) Assess and recognise the severity of a clinical presentation and a need for immediate emergency care.

(b) Diagnose and manage acute medical emergencies.

(c) Provide basic first aid.

(d) Provide immediate life support.

(e) Provide cardio-pulmonary resuscitation or direct other team members to carry out resuscitation.

17 Prescribe drugs safely, effectively and economically.

17. See GMC, *Good Practice in Prescribing Medicines;* Appendix 3, *Related documents:* 9, 10

(a) Establish an accurate drug history, covering both prescribed and other medication.

(b) Plan appropriate drug therapy for common indications, including pain and distress.

(c) Provide a safe and legal prescription.

(d) Calculate appropriate drug doses and record the outcome accurately.

(e) Provide patients with appropriate information about their medicines.

(f) Access reliable information about medicines.

(g) Detect and report adverse drug reactions.

(h) Demonstrate awareness that many patients use complementary and alternative therapies, and awareness of the existence and range of these therapies, why patients use them, and how this might affect other types of treatment that patients are receiving.

18 Carry out practical procedures safely and effectively.

(a) Be able to perform a range of diagnostic procedures, as listed in Appendix 1 and measure and record the findings.

(b) Be able to perform a range of therapeutic procedures, as listed in Appendix 1.

(c) Be able to demonstrate correct practice in general aspects of practical procedures, as listed in Appendix 1.

19 Use information effectively in a medical context.

19. See Appendix 3, *Related documents*: 43

(a) Keep accurate, legible and complete clinical records.

(b) Make effective use of computers and other information systems, including storing and retrieving information.

(c) Keep to the requirements of confidentiality and data protection legislation and codes of practice in all dealings with information.

19c. See GMC, *Confidentiality*

(d) Access information sources and use the information in relation to patient care, health promotion, giving advice and information to patients, and research and education.

19d. See GMC, *Good Medical Practice*, paragraph 12

(e) Apply the principles, method and knowledge of health informatics to medical practice.

Outcomes 3 – The doctor as a professional

20   The graduate will be able to behave according to ethical and legal principles. The graduate will be able to:

(a)   Know about and keep to the GMC's ethical guidance and standards including *Good Medical Practice*, the 'Duties of a doctor registered with the GMC' and supplementary ethical guidance which describe what is expected of all doctors registered with the GMC.

(b)   Demonstrate awareness of the clinical responsibilities and role of the doctor, making the care of the patient the first concern. Recognise the principles of patient-centred care, including self-care, and deal with patients' healthcare needs in consultation with them and, where appropriate, their relatives or carers.

(c)   Be polite, considerate, trustworthy and honest, act with integrity, maintain confidentiality, respect patients' dignity and privacy, and understand the importance of appropriate consent.

(d)   Respect all patients, colleagues and others regardless of their age, colour, culture, disability, ethnic or national origin, gender, lifestyle, marital or parental status, race, religion or beliefs, sex, sexual orientation, or social or economic status. Graduates will respect patients' right to hold religious or other beliefs, and take these into account when relevant to treatment options.

20. See GMC, *Good Medical Practice* and in particular paragraphs 56-59; Appendix 3, *Related documents:* 55, 56, 58

20d. See GMC, *Good Medical Practice*, paragraphs 7-10; GMC, *Personal beliefs;* Appendix 3, *Related documents:* 38, 46

(e) Recognise the rights and the equal value of all people and how opportunities for some people may be restricted by others' perceptions.

(f) Understand and accept the legal, moral and ethical responsibilities involved in protecting and promoting the health of individual patients, their dependants and the public – including vulnerable groups such as children, older people, people with learning disabilities and people with mental illnesses.

(g) Demonstrate knowledge of laws, and systems of professional regulation through the GMC and others, relevant to medical practice, including the ability to complete relevant certificates and legal documents and liaise with the coroner or procurator fiscal where appropriate.

21 Reflect, learn and teach others.

21. See *Good Medical Practice,* paragraphs 12-19

(a) Acquire, assess, apply and integrate new knowledge, learn to adapt to changing circumstances and ensure that patients receive the highest level of professional care.

(b) Establish the foundations for lifelong learning and continuing professional development, including a professional development portfolio containing reflections, achievements and learning needs.

(c) Continually and systematically reflect on practice and, whenever necessary, translate that reflection into action, using improvement techniques and audit appropriately – for example, by critically appraising the prescribing of others.

(d) Manage time and prioritise tasks, and work autonomously when necessary and appropriate.

(e) Recognise own personal and professional limits and seek help from colleagues and supervisors when necessary.

(f) Function effectively as a mentor and teacher including contributing to the appraisal, assessment and review of colleagues, giving effective feedback, and taking advantage of opportunities to develop these skills.

22 Learn and work effectively within a multi-professional team.

(a) Understand and respect the roles and expertise of health and social care professionals in the context of working and learning as a multi-professional team.

(b) Understand the contribution that effective interdisciplinary teamworking makes to the delivery of safe and high-quality care.

(c) Work with colleagues in ways that best serve the interests of patients, passing on information and handing over care, demonstrating flexibility, adaptability and a problem-solving approach.

22. See *Good Medical Practice*, paragraph 41; Appendix 3, *Related documents*: 17, 20

(d) Demonstrate ability to build team capacity and positive working relationships and undertake various team roles including leadership and the ability to accept leadership by others.

22d. See Appendix 3, Related documents: 42

23 Protect patients and improve care.

(a) Place patients' needs and safety at the centre of the care process.

(b) Deal effectively with uncertainty and change.

23a. See Appendix 3, Related documents: 15

(c) Understand the framework in which medicine is practised in the UK, including: the organisation, management and regulation of healthcare provision; the structures, functions and priorities of the NHS; and the roles of, and relationships between, the agencies and services involved in protecting and promoting individual and population health.

(d) Promote, monitor and maintain health and safety in the clinical setting, understanding how errors can happen in practice, applying the principles of quality assurance, clinical governance and risk management to medical practice, and understanding responsibilities within the current systems for raising concerns about safety and quality.

23d. See Appendix 3, Related documents: 57

(e) Understand and have experience of the principles and methods of improvement, including audit, adverse incident reporting and quality improvement, and how to use the results of audit to improve practice.

(f) Respond constructively to the outcomes of appraisals, performance reviews and assessments.

(g) Demonstrate awareness of the role of doctors as managers, including seeking ways to continually improve the use and prioritisation of resources.

(h) Understand the importance of, and the need to keep to, measures to prevent the spread of infection, and apply the principles of infection prevention and control.

(i) Recognise own personal health needs, consult and follow the advice of a suitably qualified professional, and protect patients from any risk posed by own health.

(j) Recognise the duty to take action if a colleague's health, performance or conduct is putting patients at risk.

Standards for the delivery of teaching, learning and assessment

24   The following paragraphs set out the standards expected for the delivery of teaching, learning and assessment in medical education. The standards are grouped under nine 'domains'. For each domain there are one or more broad 'standards'. Under these are the more technical 'criteria' by which we will judge whether medical schools are meeting these standards, and the 'evidence' used for this. The 'detailed requirements and context' expand upon the criteria, and these paragraphs contain some important principles and requirements.

25   Statements using 'must' or 'will' mean something is mandatory. Statements using 'should' may be taken into account in the quality assurance process when the GMC considers whether the overall criteria have been met.

Domain 1 – Patient safety

Standards

26 The safety of patients and their care must not be put at risk by students' duties, access to patients and supervision on placements[5] or by the performance, health or conduct of any individual student.

26. See Appendix 3, *Related documents*: 15

27 To ensure the future safety and care of patients, students who do not meet the outcomes set out in *Tomorrow's Doctors* or are otherwise not fit to practise must not be allowed to graduate with a medical degree.

27. See GMC and Medical Schools Council, *Medical students: professional values and fitness to practise*

Criteria

28 Systems and procedures will:

28. See Domain 6

(a) ensure that medical students undertake only appropriate tasks in which they are competent or are learning to be competent, and with adequate supervision

(b) identify and address immediately any concerns about patient safety arising from the education of medical students

(c) identify and address immediately any concerns about a medical student whose conduct gives cause for concern or whose health is affected to such a degree that it could harm the public, where possible through providing support to the student

(d) ensure that medical students who are not fit to practise are not allowed to graduate with a medical degree

(e) inform students, and those delivering medical education, of their responsibility to raise concerns if they identify risks to patient safety, and provide ways to do this.

Evidence

29   Evidence for this domain will include:

- medical school quality data (including inspections, reports of other visits and surveys)
- medical school guidance on fitness to practise policies and their implementation
- data from other education providers
- data from other healthcare regulators and organisations.

Detailed requirements and context

30   The medical school has a duty to ensure that systems are in place to minimise harm to anyone taking part in the training of medical students. Therefore, all those who teach, supervise, counsel, employ or work with medical students are responsible for protecting patients. The medical school must ensure that teachers and others are provided with relevant contextual information about what stage students are at in their training, what they are expected to do, and, if necessary, any concerns about a student. Medical schools must consider providing initial training in a clinical skills facility to minimise the risk to patients.

31   Although medical students may not be directly observed or supervised during all contact with the public – whether in hospitals, in general practice or in the community – there must be a general oversight of students on placement to ensure patient safety. Closer supervision will be provided when students are at lower levels of competence, ensuring that they are not put in situations where they are asked to work beyond their current competence without appropriate support.

32   The four UK health departments are responsible for deciding how students may have access to patients on NHS premises. Students are responsible for following guidance issued by the UK health departments and other organisations about their access to patients in NHS hospitals and community settings. They also need to be aware of any departmental guidance for healthcare workers which may have an effect on their practice in due course.

33   As future doctors, students have a duty to follow the guidance in *Good Medical Practice* from their first day of study and must understand the consequences if they fail to do so. In particular, students must appreciate the importance of protecting patients, even if this conflicts with their own interests or those of friends or colleagues. If students have concerns about patient safety, they must report these to their medical school. Medical schools must provide robust ways for concerns to be reported in confidence and communicate these to students.

33. See paragraph 133; also see GMC, *Good Medical Practice*

34   Students must be aware that:

- under Section 49 of the Medical Act 1983 it is an offence for a doctor to pretend to hold registration when they do not
- from the introduction of the licence to practise, it is an offence under Section 49A of the Act for a doctor to pretend to hold a licence when they do not.

35   Clinical tutors and supervisors[6] must make honest and objective judgements when appraising or assessing the performance of students, including those they have supervised or trained. Patients may be put at risk if a student is described as competent without having reached or maintained a satisfactory standard.

36   Guidance is given in the joint GMC and Medical Schools Council publication *Medical students: professional values and fitness to practise* about how medical schools should handle concerns about a medical student's performance, health or conduct. The most appropriate form for a medical school's fitness to practise procedures will be decided by the medical school, taking into account the university's structure and statutes. But they should include provision for immediate steps to be taken to investigate any concerns to identify whether they are well-founded and to protect patients. There should also be a flow of information between medical schools and other education providers to ensure that clinical tutors and supervisors are appropriately informed.

36. See paragraphs 145-147; also see GMC and Medical Schools Council, *Medical students: professional values and fitness to practise*

37   From the introduction of the licence to practise, a student awarded a recognised PMQ is eligible for provisional registration with a licence to practise with the GMC, subject to their fitness to practise not being impaired. By awarding a medical degree, the awarding body[7] is confirming that the medical graduate is fit to practise as a Foundation Year One doctor to the high standards that we have set in our guidance to the medical profession, *Good Medical Practice*. Therefore, university medical schools have a responsibility to the public, to employers and to the profession to ensure that only those students who are fit to practise as doctors are allowed to complete the curriculum and gain provisional registration with a licence to practise. This responsibility covers both the thorough assessment of students' knowledge, skills and behaviour towards the end of the course, and appropriate consideration of any concerns about a student's performance, health or conduct.

37. See Domain 5; also see GMC, *Good Medical Practice*

Domain 2 – Quality assurance, review and evaluation

Standard

38   The quality of medical education programmes will be monitored, reviewed and evaluated in a systematic way.

Criteria

39   The medical school will have a clear framework or plan for how it organises quality management and quality control, including who is responsible for this.

40   Management systems will be in place to plan and monitor undergraduate medical education (including admissions, courses, placements, student supervision and support, assessment and resources) to ensure that it meets required standards of quality.

41   The medical school will have agreements with providers of each clinical or vocational placement, and will have systems to monitor the quality of teaching and facilities on placements.

42   The medical school will produce regular reports about different stages or aspects of the curriculum and its delivery, and these will be considered at appropriate management levels of the medical school. There will be systems to plan, implement and review enhancements or changes to the curriculum or its delivery.

43   Quality data will include:

(a) evaluations by students and data from medical school
teachers and other education providers about placements,
resources and assessment outcomes

(b) feedback from patients

(c) feedback from employers about the preparedness
of graduates.

44   Concerns about, or risks to, the quality of any aspect of
undergraduate medical education will be identified and
managed quickly and effectively.

Evidence

45   The evidence for this domain will include:

- university and medical school quality assurance
documentation, including policies, handbooks and
minutes of meetings
- documentation about expected standards of curriculum
delivery, including placement agreements with other
education providers
- monitoring reports and reports of inspections or visits
- quality-control data including student evaluations.

Detailed requirements and context

46 General guidance on quality assurance is given in the Quality Assurance Agency (QAA) *Code of practice for the assurance of academic quality and standards in higher education.* Medical schools should draw on this when designing systems and procedures for quality assurance, management and control.

47 Quality management policies and procedures at a medical school will vary according to the university's structure and statutes. But these must include clear information about roles and responsibilities, committee structures, lines of reporting and authority, and the timing of monitoring reports and reviews.

48 Apart from the medical school officers and committees, all education providers of clinical placements, and all clinical tutors and supervisors, students, employers and patients should be involved in quality management and control processes. Their roles must be defined and information made available to them about this.

46. See Appendix 3, *Related documents*: 60

49 Quality management must cover all aspects of undergraduate medical education, not just teaching. This covers planning, monitoring and the identification and resolution of problems, and includes the following areas:

- admission to medical school
- the learning experience (including induction, teaching, supervision, placements, curriculum)
- appraisal of, and feedback to, students
- pastoral and academic support for students
- assessment of students
- educational resources and capacity (including funding and facilities).

50 As part of quality management, there must be agreements in place with providers of each clinical or vocational placement. These agreements should set out roles and responsibilities, the learning objectives for the placement, and arrangements to ensure that medical students have appropriate learning opportunities to meet the learning outcomes.

50. See paragraphs 157, 165.

51 There must be procedures in place to check the quality of teaching, learning and assessment, including that in clinical/vocational placements, and to ensure that standards are being maintained. These must be monitored through a number of different systems, including student and patient feedback, and reviews of teaching by peers. Appraisals should cover teaching responsibilities for all relevant consultant, academic and other staff, whether or not employed by the university.

52　There must also be systems in place to check the quality and management of educational resources and their capacity, and to ensure that standards are maintained. These must include the management and allocation of funding, clear plans for the planning and management of facilities, and monitoring of student numbers on placements to prevent overcrowding.

53　Any problems identified through gathering and analysing quality-control data should be addressed as soon as possible. It should be clear who is responsible for this. There should also be documentation covering:

- the actions taken
- the feedback given to students and staff on what is being done
- how the problems were resolved.

54　Given the importance of assessment, including placement-based assessments, there must be specific quality-control standards and systems in place to ensure the assessments are 'fit for purpose'.

54. See Domain 5

55　The quality assurance system should ensure that, through the regular reporting upwards on all aspects of undergraduate medical education, the medical school can keep these under constant review, and introduce changes and enhancements. This will include, but should not be limited to, the reviews of faculties, schools or degree programmes prescribed by university procedures.

Domain 3 – Equality, diversity and opportunity

Standard

56   Undergraduate medical education must be fair and based on principles of equality.

56. See Appendix 3, *Related documents*: 44

Criteria

57   The medical school will have policies which are aimed at ensuring that all applicants and students are treated fairly and with equality of opportunity, regardless of their diverse backgrounds.

58   Staff will receive training on equality and diversity to ensure they are aware of their responsibilities and the issues that need to be taken into account when undertaking their roles in the medical school.

59   Reasonable adjustments will be made for students with disabilities in accordance with current legislation and guidance.

59. See GMC and others, *Gateways to the professions: advising medical schools: encouraging disabled students*; Appendix 3, *Related documents*: 30, 45

60   The medical school will routinely collect and analyse data about equality and diversity issues to ensure that policies are being implemented and any concerns are identified.

61   The medical school will act promptly over any concerns about equality and diversity, implementing and monitoring any changes to policy and practice.

Evidence

62   Evidence for this domain will include:

- medical school policies and action plans about equality and diversity
- information about staff training in equality and diversity, including data on attendance/compliance
- monitoring data about student applications: evidence of addressing equality and diversity matters within admissions processes, progression, assessment and arrangements made for supervision, covering sex, race, disability, sexual orientation, religion or belief, gender identity and age
- information about 'reasonable adjustments' made for students with disabilities and the procedures in place to review the effectiveness of the adjustments
- reports and minutes of meetings.

Detailed requirements and context

63   This domain is concerned with ensuring that students and applicants to medical schools are treated fairly and impartially, with equality of opportunity, regardless of factors that are irrelevant to their selection and progress. It is also concerned with encouraging diversity within the student population to reflect modern society.

64   Specific advice on disabled applicants and students is given in the *Gateways* guidance. Medical schools should have policies on disability which take into account this guidance, relevant legislation and good practice elsewhere. These should cover the assessment of an applicant's ability to meet the 'outcomes for graduates', and the provision of reasonable adjustments and support for a student. Schools should consult each individual concerned to identify the most appropriate adjustments and have them in place before the student's course begins. Schools should review the effectiveness of the adjustments once the student has had time to benefit from their introduction.

64. See GMC and others, *Gateways to the professions: advising medical schools: encouraging disabled studentss*; Appendix 3, *Related documents*: 27

65   Medical schools should have clear policies, guidance and action plans for tackling discrimination and harassment, and for promoting equality and diversity generally. Medical schools should ensure that these meet the current relevant legal requirements of their country and that they are made available to students.

66   Medical schools' policies for the training, conduct and assessment of students should have regard for the variety of cultural, social and religious backgrounds of students, while maintaining consistency in educational and professional standards.

67 Medical schools should have clear guidance on any areas where a student's culture or religion may conflict with usual practice or rules, including when on placements – for example, dress codes or the scheduling of classes and examinations.

68 Monitoring data must be collected, used and stored in keeping with current legislation and guidance about data protection, confidentiality and privacy.

69 All providers of education and work experience must demonstrate their commitment to equality and diversity.

70 An important part of ensuring equality and diversity is the support provided to students.

70. See Domain 6

Domain 4 – Student selection

Standard

71 Processes for student selection will be open, objective and fair.

71. See Appendix 3, *Related documents*: 26

Criteria

72 The medical school will publish information about the admission system, including guidance about the selection process and the basis on which places at the school will be offered.

73 Selection criteria will take account of the personal and academic qualities needed in a doctor as set out in *Good Medical Practice* and capacity to achieve the outcomes set out in *Tomorrow's Doctors*.

73. See GMC, *Good Medical Practice*; Appendix 3, *Related documents*: 58

74 Selection processes will be valid, reliable and objective.

75 Those responsible for student selection will include people with a range of expertise and knowledge. They will be trained to apply selection guidelines consistently and fairly. They will also be trained to be able to promote equality and diversity (people's different backgrounds and circumstances) and follow current equal opportunities legislation and good practice, including that covering disabled applicants.

75. See Appendix 3, *Related documents*: 27

76 Students admitted will pass any health and other checks (such as criminal record checks) required by the medical school's fitness to practise policy. The purpose and implications of each of these checks, and the points at which they are made, should be made clear to applicants and students.

76. See Appendix 3, *Related documents*: 29

Evidence

77 Evidence for this domain will include:

- information about medical school selection processes
- data about applicants and selected students
- minutes of committees and reports.

Detailed requirements and context

78 Medical schools should base their policies and procedures on relevant guidance, recognised best practice, and research into effective, reliable and valid selection processes which can have the confidence of applicants and the public.

79 Medical schools should also take account of relevant legislation and the *Gateways* guidance in their student selection processes. This includes the requirement to make reasonable adjustments for students with disabilities where the disability would not prevent the applicant from meeting the outcomes for graduates. Schools should be wary of not offering a place on the basis of a judgement about hypothetical barriers to achievement and employment specifically associated with an applicant's disability.

79. See GMC and others, *Gateways to the professions: advising medical schools: encouraging disabled students*

80   The assessment of any risks associated with an applicant's fitness to practise in relation to their health or conduct should be separated from other processes of selection.

Domain 5 – Design and delivery of the curriculum, including assessment

Standard

81   The curriculum must be designed, delivered and assessed to ensure that graduates demonstrate all the 'outcomes for graduates' specified in *Tomorrow's Doctors*.

Criteria

82   A clear curriculum plan will set out how the 'outcomes for graduates' will be met across the programme as a whole. The curriculum will include opportunities for students to exercise choice in areas of interest.

83   The curriculum will be structured to provide a balance of learning opportunities and to integrate the learning of basic and clinical sciences, enabling students to link theory and practice.

84 The curriculum will include practical experience of working with patients throughout all years, increasing in duration and responsibility so that graduates are prepared for their responsibilities as provisionally registered doctors. It will provide enough structured clinical placements to enable students to demonstrate the 'outcomes for graduates' across a range of clinical specialties, including at least one Student Assistantship[8] period.

84. See Appendix 3, *Related documents:* 28

85 Students will have regular feedback on their performance.

86 All the 'outcomes for graduates' will be assessed at appropriate points during the curriculum, ensuring that only students who meet these outcomes are permitted to graduate. Assessments will be fit for purpose – that is: valid, reliable, generalisable,[9] feasible and fair.

87 Students will receive timely and accurate guidance about assessments, including assessment format, length and range of content, marking schedule and contribution to overall grade.

88 Examiners and assessors will be appropriately selected, trained, supported and appraised.

89 There will be systems in place to set appropriate standards for assessments to decide whether students have achieved the curriculum outcomes.

90 Assessment criteria will be consistent with the requirements for competence standards set out in disability discrimination legislation. Reasonable adjustments will be provided to help students with disabilities meet these competence standards. Although reasonable adjustments cannot be made to the competence standards themselves, reasonable adjustments should be made to enable a disabled person to meet a competence standard.

Evidence

91 Evidence for this domain will include and principally be:

- the curriculum plan
- schemes of assessment
- supporting documentation, including the proportion of the curriculum devoted to Student Selected Components (SSCs).

There must also be supplementary information about the delivery of teaching and clinical placements, the operation of assessments and evaluations from students.

Detailed requirements and context

Curriculum design and structure:

Criteria, paragraph 82: A clear curriculum plan will set out how the 'outcomes for graduates' will be met across the programme as a whole. The curriculum will include opportunities for students to exercise choice in areas of interest.

92   It is for each medical school to design its own curriculum to suit its own circumstances, consistent with *Tomorrow's Doctors*. Both curriculum design and delivery must take into account modern educational theory and current research.

93   The overall curriculum must allow students to meet the outcomes specified in the first part of *Tomorrow's Doctors*. This is to ensure that graduates have the necessary knowledge, skills and behaviours to practise as a provisionally registered doctor. Medical schools must demonstrate the way in which these outcomes are met.

94   The curriculum must allow for student choice for a minimum of 10% of course time.

95   SSCs must be an integral part of the curriculum, enabling students to demonstrate mandatory competences while allowing choice in studying an area of particular interest to them.

96　The purpose of SSCs is the intellectual development of students through exploring in depth a subject of their choice.

97　SSC learning outcomes must be mapped to outcomes in *Tomorrow's Doctors*, and contained within the assessment blueprint for the programme, thus helping to make SSCs transparently relevant and clarify how SSCs contribute to the programme.

98　The assessment of these elements of the curriculum must be integrated into the overall assessment of students.

99　Information on the extent and nature of choice available in each SSC, and details on how they will be assessed and contribute to the overall assessment of students, must be publicly available for prospective and current students.

Teaching and learning:

> **Criteria, paragraph 83:** *The curriculum will be structured to provide a balance of learning opportunities and to integrate the learning of basic and clinical sciences, enabling students to link theory and practice.*

100　Students must have different teaching and learning opportunities that should balance teaching in large groups with small groups. They must have practical classes and opportunities for self-directed learning. Medical schools should take advantage of new technologies, including simulation, to deliver teaching.

101 The structure and content of courses and clinical attachments should integrate learning about basic medical sciences and clinical sciences. Students should, wherever possible, learn in a context relevant to medical practice, and revisit topics at different stages and levels to reinforce understanding and develop skills and behaviours.

101. See Appendix 3, *Related documents:* 17, 20

102 Medical schools must ensure that students work with and learn from other health and social care professionals and students. Opportunities should also be provided for students to learn with other health and social care students, including the use of simulated training environments with audiovisual recording and behavioural debriefing. This will help students understand the importance of teamwork in providing care.

Clinical placements and experience:

Criteria, paragraph 84: The curriculum will include practical experience of working with patients throughout all years, increasing in duration and responsibility so that graduates are prepared for their responsibilities as provisionally registered doctors. It will provide enough structured clinical placements to enable students to demonstrate the 'outcomes for graduates' across a range of clinical specialties, including at least one Student Assistantship[8] period.

103   The curriculum must include early and continuing contact with patients. Experiential learning in clinical settings, both real and simulated, is important to ensure graduates' preparedness for Foundation Year One (F1) training. Over the curriculum it should increase in complexity, and the level of involvement and responsibility of the student should also increase.

104   From the start, students must have opportunities to interact with people from a range of social, cultural, and ethnic backgrounds and with a range of disabilities, illnesses or conditions. Such contact with patients encourages students to gain confidence in communicating with a wide range of people, and can help develop their ability to take patients' histories and examine patients.

105   The involvement of patients in teaching must be consistent with *Good Medical Practice* and other guidance on consent published by the GMC.

105. See GMC, *Good Medical Practice*; GMC, *Consent: patients and doctors making decisions together*

106 Clinical placements must be planned and structured to give each student experience across a range of specialties, rather than relying entirely upon this arising by chance. These specialties must include medicine, obstetrics and gynaecology, paediatrics, surgery, psychiatry and general practice. Placements should reflect the changing patterns of healthcare and must provide experience in a variety of environments including hospitals, general practices and community medical services. Within each placement there must be a plan of which outcomes will be covered, how this will be delivered, and the ways in which students' performance will be assessed and students given feedback.

106. See Domain 2

107 Medical schools should ensure that appropriate arrangements are made for students with disabilities on placements. Students should be encouraged to feed back to the medical school on their experience, for example, in relation to the provision of reasonable adjustments, guidance and pastoral support, and the working culture. Medical schools should ensure appropriate feedback is communicated to the placement provider and that they intervene, where appropriate, to ensure students receive the support they require.

108 During the later years of the curriculum, students should have the opportunity to become increasingly competent in their clinical skills and in planning patient care. They should have a defined role in medical teams, subject to considerations of patient safety, and this should become more central as their education continues.

108. See Domain 1

109 In the final year, students must use practical and clinical skills, rehearsing their eventual responsibilities as an F1 doctor. These must include making recommendations for the prescription of drugs and managing acutely ill patients under the supervision of a qualified doctor. This should take the form of one or more Student Assistantships in which a student, assisting a junior doctor and under supervision, undertakes most of the duties of an F1 doctor.[10]

110 Students must be properly prepared for their first allocated F1 post. Separate from and following their Student Assistantship, they should, wherever practicable, have a period working with the F1 who is in the post they will take up when they graduate. This 'shadowing' period allows students to become familiar with the facilities available, the working environment and the working patterns expected of them, and to get to know their colleagues. It also provides an opportunity to develop working relationships with the clinical and educational supervisors they will work with in the future. It should consist of 'protected time' involving tasks that enable students to use their medical knowledge and expertise in a working environment, distinct from the general induction sessions provided for new employees and Foundation Programme trainees. The 'shadowing' period should normally last at least one week and take place as close to the point of employment as possible.

Feedback and assessment:

Criteria, paragraph 85: Students will have regular feedback on their performance.

Criteria, paragraph 86: All the 'outcomes for graduates' will be assessed at appropriate points during the curriculum, ensuring that only students who meet these outcomes are permitted to graduate. Assessments will be fit for purpose – that is: valid, reliable, generalisable,[9] feasible and fair.

Criteria, paragraph 87: Students will receive timely and accurate guidance about assessments, including assessment format, length and range of content, marking schedule and contribution to overall grade.

Criteria, paragraph 88: Examiners and assessors will be appropriately selected, trained, supported and appraised.

Criteria, paragraph 89: There will be systems in place to set appropriate standards for assessments to decide whether students have achieved the curriculum outcomes.

Criteria, paragraph 90: Assessment criteria will be consistent with the requirements for competence standards set out in disability discrimination legislation. Reasonable adjustments will be provided to help students with disabilities meet these competence standards. Although reasonable adjustments cannot be made to the competence standards themselves, reasonable adjustments should be made to enable a disabled person to meet a competence standard.

111   Students must receive regular information about their
development and progress. This should include feedback on
both formative and summative assessments. Clinical logbooks
and personal portfolios, which allow students to identify
strengths and weaknesses and to focus their learning, can
provide this information. Using these will emphasise the
importance of maintaining a portfolio of evidence of
achievement, which will be necessary once they have become
doctors and their licence to practise is regularly revalidated.
All doctors, other health and social care workers, patients
and carers who come into contact with the student should
have an opportunity to provide constructive feedback about
their performance. Feedback about performance in
assessments helps to identify strengths and weaknesses,
both in students and in the curriculum, and this allows
changes to be made.

112   Medical schools must ensure that all graduates have achieved
all the outcomes set out in *Tomorrow's Doctors*, that is:

- each of the five outcomes under 'The doctor as a scholar
  and a scientist'
- each of the seven outcomes under 'The doctor as a
  practitioner'
- each of the four outcomes under 'The doctor as
  a professional'
- every practical procedure listed in Appendix 1.

This must involve summative assessments during the course that cumulatively demonstrate achievement of each outcome. The medical school must have schemes of assessment that map the outcomes to each assessment event and type, across an appropriate range of disciplines and specialties ('blueprinting'). Students' knowledge, skills and professional behaviour must be assessed. There must be a description of how individual assessments and examinations contribute to the overall assessment of curricular outcomes, which must be communicated to staff and students.

113   Assessments must be designed and delivered to provide a valid and reliable judgement of a student's performance. This means that methods of assessment must measure what they set out to measure, and do so in a fair and consistent way. A range of assessment techniques should be used, with medical schools deciding which are most appropriate for their curriculum.

114   Students must have guidance about what is expected of them in any examination or assessment. No question format will be used in a summative assessment that has not previously been used in a formative assessment of the student concerned.

115   Examiners[11] must be trained to carry out their role and to apply the medical school's assessment criteria consistently. They should have guidelines for marking assessments, which indicate how performance against targeted curricular outcomes should be rewarded.

116 Medical schools must have mechanisms to ensure comparability of standards with other institutions and to share good practice. The mechanisms must cover the appointment of external examiners. The duties and powers of external examiners must be clearly set out.

117 Medical schools must have appropriate methods for setting standards in assessments to decide whether students have achieved the 'outcomes for graduates'. There must be no compensatory mechanism which would allow students to graduate without having demonstrated competence in all the outcomes.

118 Those responsible for assessment must keep to relevant legislation and aim to apply good practice relating to the assessment of those with a disability. Medical schools should also take account of the *Gateways* guidance.

119 Medical schools should be guided by the QAA *Code of practice for the assurance of academic quality and standards in higher education*.

118. See GMC and others, *Gateways to the professions: advising medical schools: encouraging disabled students*

119. See Appendix 3, *Related documents*: 60

120 Medical schools must use evidence from research into best practice to decide how to plan and organise their assessments: from blueprinting and choosing valid and reliable methods to standard-setting and operational matters. Medical schools must be able to explain clearly their schemes of assessment and demonstrate a wide understanding of them among their staff. Medical schools must therefore have staff with expertise in assessment or access to such staff in other institutions to advise on good practice and train staff involved in assessment.

121 Undergraduate medical education is part of a continuum of education and training which continues through postgraduate training and continuing professional development. While it is essential that the outcomes are achieved by all graduates, medical schools should also make arrangements so that graduates' areas of relative weakness are fed into their Foundation Programme portfolios so they can be reviewed by the educational supervisor. This information should draw on assessments in relation to the outcomes and include graduating transcripts.

Domain 6 – Support and development of students, teachers and the local faculty

Standard

122 Students must receive both academic and general guidance and support, including when they are not progressing well or otherwise causing concern. Everyone teaching or supporting students must themselves be supported, trained and appraised.

Criteria

123 Students will have comprehensive guidance about the curriculum, their placements, what is expected of them and how they will be assessed.

124 Students will have appropriate support for their academic and general welfare needs and will be given information about these support networks.

125 Students will have access to career advice, and opportunities to explore different careers in medicine. Appropriate alternative qualification pathways will be available to those who decide to leave medicine.

126 Students will be encouraged to look after their own health and given information about their responsibilities in this respect as a trainee doctor. They will feel confident in seeking appropriate advice, support and treatment in a confidential and supportive environment.

127 Medical schools will have robust and fair procedures to deal with students who are causing concern on academic and/or non-academic grounds. Fitness to practise arrangements and procedures will take account of the guidance issued by the GMC and the Medical Schools Council. Students must have clear information about these procedures.

127. See GMC and Medical Schools Council, *Medical students: professional values and fitness to practise*

128 Everyone involved in educating medical students will be appropriately selected, trained, supported and appraised.

Evidence

129 Evidence for this domain will include:

- ◼ medical school documentation about student support arrangements
- ◼ regulations and procedures
- ◼ documentation about support and training provided to staff and other education providers
- ◼ inspection reports
- ◼ medical school quality management reports.

Detailed requirements and context

Academic and pastoral support and guidance:

Criteria, paragraph 123: *Students will have comprehensive guidance about the curriculum, their placements, what is expected of them and how they will be assessed.*

Criteria, paragraph 124: *Students will have appropriate support for their academic and general welfare needs and will be given information about these support networks.*

Criteria, paragraph 125: *Students will have access to career advice, and opportunities to explore different careers in medicine. Appropriate alternative qualification pathways will be available to those who decide to leave medicine.*

130   Medical schools must give students comprehensive guidance about the curriculum and how their performance will be assessed. This must include:

- information about the objectives of clinical placements and how they are assessed
- briefing about practical arrangements for assessments
- the medical school's policies on cheating, plagiarism and the importance of probity.

Students should also be able to get academic advice and guidance from identified members of staff if they need it in a particular subject.

131 Students must have appropriate support for their academic and general welfare needs at all stages. Medical schools must produce information about the support networks available, including named contacts for students with problems. Students taking SSCs that are taught in other departments or by other medical schools, and those on clinical attachments or on electives, must have access to appropriate support.

132 Guidance and support in making reasonable adjustments can be found in the *Gateways* guidance and should also be sought from an appropriate member of staff, such as a disability officer. Implementing reasonable adjustments promptly and reviewing their effectiveness may remedy the difficulties faced by the student. It is important that the medical school gives sufficient time for the student to reap the benefit of the adjustment (and receive the necessary training to use the adjustment, where required) before reviewing the situation.

132. See GMC and others, *Gateways to the professions: advising medical schools: encouraging disabled students*; GMC and Medical Schools Council, *Medical students: professional values and fitness to practise*, paragraph 48.

133 Support and guidance must be provided for students who raise concerns about the health or conduct of anyone else, in order to protect them from victimisation. The process for raising such concerns must be made clear to students.

133. See Appendix 3, *Related documents*: 18

134 Schools must have a careers guidance strategy. Generic resources should include an outline of career paths in medicine and the postgraduate specialties, as well as guidance on application forms and processes. Specific guidance should be provided for personalised career planning. The careers strategy should be developed and updated with the local postgraduate deanery.

135 A small number of students may discover that they have made a wrong career choice. Medical schools must make sure that these students, whose academic and non-academic performance is not in question, are able to gain an alternative degree or to transfer to another degree course.

136 Students who do not meet the necessary standards in terms of demonstrating appropriate knowledge, skills and behaviour should be advised of alternative careers to follow.

Students' health:

Criteria, paragraph 126: Students will be encouraged to look after their own health and given information about their responsibilities in this respect as a trainee doctor. They will feel confident in seeking appropriate advice, support and treatment in a confidential and supportive environment.

137 It is important to differentiate between disability and ill-health in relation to fitness to practise. Having an impairment does not mean that a person is in a permanent state of poor health.

137. See GMC and others, *Gateways to the professions: advising medical schools: encouraging disabled students,* section 3.2

138 Medical schools must stress to students the importance of looking after their own health, encourage them to register with a general practitioner and emphasise that they may not be able to assess their own health accurately. They must tell students about the occupational health services, including counselling, that are available to them.

139 Medical students who may be experiencing difficulties due to a disability, illness or condition should be encouraged to get appropriate help so that they might receive informed advice and support, including reasonable adjustments where appropriate. Students who misuse drugs or alcohol should also be provided with appropriate advice and support.

140 *Good Medical Practice* requires doctors to take responsibility for their own health in the interests of public safety, and medical students should also follow this guidance. Students should protect patients, colleagues and themselves by being immunised against serious communicable diseases where vaccines are available. If a student knows that they have a serious condition which could be passed on to patients, or that their judgement or performance could be significantly affected by a condition or illness (or its treatment), they must take and follow advice from a consultant in occupational health or from another suitably qualified doctor on whether, and in what ways, their clinical contact with patients should be altered. Students should not rely on their own assessment of the risk to patients.

140. See GMC, *Good Medical Practice*

141   Guidance on the responsibilities of students and the medical
school is in the *Medical School Charter*, produced jointly by
the Medical Schools Council and the Medical Students
Committee of the British Medical Association.

141. See
Appendix 3,
*Related
documents*: 19

142   Medical schools and students must also be aware of the
four UK health departments' guidance on exposure-prone
procedures.

143   Medical students who are ill have the same rights to
confidentiality as other patients. Doctors providing medical
care for students must consider their duties under the GMC's
Confidentiality guidance. Passing on personal information
without permission may be justified if failure to do so may
result in death or serious harm to the patient or to others.
Doctors should not pass on information without the student's
permission, unless the risk to patients is so serious that it
outweighs the student's rights to privacy. They must
remember that students will be in close contact with patients
from an early stage of their training.

143. See GMC,
Confidentiality

144   Doctors providing medical care for students should consult
an experienced colleague, or get advice from a professional
organisation, if they are not sure whether passing on
information without a medical student's permission is
justified.

Student progression and fitness to practise procedures:

Criteria, paragraph 127: Medical schools will have robust and fair procedures to deal with students who are causing concern on academic and or non-academic grounds. Fitness to practise arrangements and procedures will take account of the guidance issued by the GMC and MSC. Students must have clear information about these procedures.

145   Medical schools must provide appropriate support, advice and adjustments. They must also have robust and fair arrangements and procedures, including an appeals process, to deal with students who are causing concern – either on academic or non-academic grounds, including ill-health or misconduct. Medical schools must tell students about these arrangements and procedures so that they understand their rights and obligations. The medical school should decide on the most appropriate form of procedures, taking into account its statutes and circumstances.

145. See GMC and Medical Schools Council, *Medical students: professional values and fitness to practise*

146   If a student's fitness to practise is called into question because of their behaviour or their health, the medical school's arrangements must take account of the joint GMC and MSC guidance: *Medical students: professional values and fitness to practise.* The arrangements should cover both informal and formal procedures, and include clear policies on disclosure of information and evidence to students, to staff and outside the medical school, such as to deaneries and the GMC.

147 The GMC can agree arrangements for disabled graduates so that they are not disadvantaged unfairly by their disability when participating in F1 training, under Section 10A(2)(f) of the Medical Act 1983. Medical schools should contact us at the earliest opportunity should they consider that such arrangements may become necessary for any of their students. The educational aspects of postgraduate medical training are subject to an anticipatory duty to make reasonable adjustments for disabled trainees. It is expected that doctors with a range of disabilities and health conditions should be able to meet the outcomes for F1.

Support for educators:

Criteria, paragraph 128: Everyone involved in educating medical students will be appropriately selected, trained, supported and appraised.

148 Medical schools must make sure that everyone involved in educating medical students has the necessary knowledge and skills for their role. This includes teachers, trainers, clinical supervisors and assessors in the medical school or with other education providers. They should also make sure that these people understand *Tomorrow's Doctors* and put it into practice. The medical school must ensure that appropriate training is provided to these people to carry out their role, and that staff-development programmes promote teaching and assessment skills. All staff (including those from other education providers) should take part in such programmes.

149 Every doctor who comes into contact with medical students should recognise the importance of role models in developing appropriate behaviours towards patients, colleagues and others. Doctors with particular responsibility for teaching students must develop the skills and practices of a competent teacher and must make sure that students are properly supervised.

Domain 7 – Management of teaching, learning and assessment

Standard
150 Education must be planned and managed using processes which show who is responsible for each process or stage.

Criteria
151 A management plan at medical school level will show who is responsible for curriculum planning, teaching, learning and assessment at each stage of the undergraduate programme, and how they manage these processes.

152 Teachers from the medical school and other education providers will be closely involved in curriculum management, represented at medical school level and responsible for managing their own areas of the programme.

153 Employers of graduates, and bodies responsible for their continuing training, will be closely involved in curriculum planning and management.

Evidence

154 Evidence for this domain will include:

- medical school policies
- management plans
- agreements with providers of clinical or vocational placements.

Detailed requirements and context

155 Medical schools should have supervisory structures that involve individuals with an appropriate range of expertise and knowledge. Lines of authority and responsibility must be set out. This will allow medical schools to plan curricula and associated assessments, put them into practice and review them. Having people with educational expertise in a medical education unit can help this process.

156 It must be clear who is responsible for the day-to-day management of parts of the curriculum, such as courses and placements, and how those responsible report to higher management levels. Medical school teachers and other education providers and their staff should be involved in managing their own areas of the curriculum, and should be represented on medical school committees and groups.

157 The medical school must have agreements with the other education providers who contribute to the delivery of the curriculum. These should specify the contribution, including teaching, resources and the relevant curriculum outcomes, and how these contributions combine to satisfy the requirements set out in *Tomorrow's Doctors*.

158 The four UK health departments have the role of ensuring that NHS organisations work with medical schools so that students receive appropriate clinical training.

Domain 8 – Educational resources and capacity

Standard
159 The educational facilities and infrastructure must be appropriate to deliver the curriculum.

Criteria
160 Students will have access to appropriate learning resources and facilities including libraries, computers, lecture theatres, seminar rooms and appropriate environments to develop and improve their knowledge, skills and behaviour.

161 Facilities will be supported by a facilities management plan which provides for regular review of the fitness for purpose of the facilities with recommendations and improvements made where appropriate. When reviewing facilities, medical schools should include their suitability for students with disabilities.

162 There will be enough staff from appropriate disciplines, and with the necessary skills and experience, to deliver teaching and support students' learning.

Evidence

163 Evidence for this domain will include:

- medical schools' facilities management plans
- data on facilities usage
- internal quality management reports.

Detailed requirements and context

164 Medical schools must have a plan for the management of resources and facilities. This plan should map to the curriculum to ensure that resources and facilities are effectively used. The plan should also provide for the regular review of facilities to ensure they are still appropriate. Facilities should be accessible for students and others with a disability. Students must be able to comment about the facilities and suggest new resources that should be provided, and schools should consider these comments and feed back their conclusions.

165 The four UK health departments have a duty to make facilities in NHS hospitals and other premises available for students to receive clinical training. Resources will be covered in the agreements between medical schools and other education providers who contribute to the delivery of the curriculum. The agreements will set out the process by which the medical schools can be clear about the allocation of the financial resources received to support undergraduate medical education.

166 Students must have opportunities to develop and improve their clinical and practical skills in an appropriate environment (where they are supported by teachers) before they use these skills in clinical situations. Skills laboratories and centres provide an excellent setting for this training.

167 Learning in an environment that is committed to care, based on evidence and research, can help medical students to understand the importance of developing research and audit skills to improve their practice. It also helps to make sure that those responsible for their learning are aware of current developments in clinical theory and practice.

Domain 9 – Outcomes

Standards

168 The outcomes for graduates of undergraduate medical education in the UK are set out in *Tomorrow's Doctors*. All medical students will demonstrate these outcomes before graduating from medical school.

168. See Appendix 3, *Related documents*: 13, 14

169 The medical schools must track the impact of the outcomes for graduates and the standards for delivery as set out in *Tomorrow's Doctors* against the knowledge, skills and behaviour of students and graduates.

Criteria

170 The programme of undergraduate medical education employs a curriculum which is demonstrated to meet the outcomes for graduates.

171 The programme requires that graduates are able to demonstrate the outcomes.

172 Quality management will involve the collection and use of information about the progression of students. It will also involve the collection and use of information about the subsequent progression of graduates in relation to the Foundation Programme and postgraduate training, and in respect of any determinations by the GMC.

173 Students must have access to analysis of the results of assessments and examinations at the school.

Evidence

174 Evidence for this domain will include:

- medical school quality data – including data from staff, other education providers and students, and data concerning the progression of graduates
- documentation that demonstrates the use of this information in quality management.

Appendix 1 –
Practical procedures for graduates

Diagnostic procedures

Procedure	Description in lay terms
1. Measuring body temperature	... using an appropriate recording device.
2. Measuring pulse rate and blood pressure	... using manual techniques and automatic electronic devices.
3. Transcutaneous monitoring of oxygen saturation	Applying, and taking readings from, an electronic device which measures the amount of oxygen in the patient's blood.
4. Venepuncture	Inserting a needle into a patient's vein to take a sample of blood for testing, or to give an injection into the vein.
5. Managing blood samples correctly	Making sure that blood samples are placed in the correct containers, and that these are labelled correctly and sent to the laboratory promptly and in the correct way. Taking measures to prevent spilling and contamination.
6. Taking blood cultures	Taking samples of venous blood to test for the growth of infectious organisms in the blood. Requires special blood containers and laboratory procedures.
7. Measuring blood glucose	Measuring the concentration of glucose in the patient's blood at the bedside, using appropriate equipment and interpreting the results.
8. Managing an electrocardiograph (ECG) monitor	Setting up a continuous recording of the electrical activity of the heart. Ensuring the recorder is functioning correctly, and interpreting the tracing.

Diagnostic procedures (continued)

Procedure	Description in lay terms
9. Performing and interpreting a 12-lead electrocardiograph (ECG)	Recording a full, detailed tracing of the electrical activity of the heart, using a machine recorder (electrocardiograph). Interpreting the recording for signs of heart disease.
10. Basic respiratory function tests	Carrying out basic tests to see how well the patient's lungs are working (for example, how much air they can breathe out in one second).
11. Urinalysis using Multistix	Testing a sample of urine for abnormal contents, such as blood or protein. The urine is applied to a plastic strip with chemicals which change colour in response to specific abnormalities.
12. Advising patients on how to collect a mid-stream urine specimen	Obtaining a sample of urine from a patient, usually to check for the presence of infection, using a method which reduces the risk of contamination by skin bacteria.
13. Taking nose, throat and skin swabs	Using the correct technique to apply sterile swabs to the nose, throat and skin.
14. Nutritional assessment	Making an assessment of the patient's state of nutrition. This includes an evaluation of their diet; their general physical condition; and measurement of height, weight and body mass index.
15. Pregnancy testing	Performing a test of the urine to detect hormones which indicate that the patient is pregnant.

Therapeutic procedures

Procedure	Description in lay terms
16. Administering oxygen	Allowing the patient to breathe a higher concentration of oxygen than normal, via a face mask or other equipment.
17. Establishing peripheral intravenous access and setting up an infusion; use of infusion devices	Puncturing a patient's vein in order to insert an indwelling plastic tube (known as a 'cannula'), to allow fluids to be infused into the vein (a 'drip'). Connecting the tube to a source of fluid. Appropriate choice of fluids and their doses. Correct use of electronic devices which drive and regulate the rate of fluid administration.
18. Making up drugs for parenteral administration	Preparing medicines in a form suitable for injection into the patient's vein. May involve adding the drug to a volume of fluid to make up the correct concentration for injection.
19. Dosage and administration of insulin and use of sliding scales	Calculating how many units of insulin a patient requires, what strength of insulin solution to use, and how it should be given (for example, into the skin, or into a vein). Use of a 'sliding scale' which links the number of units to the patient's blood glucose measurement at the time.
20. Subcutaneous and intramuscular injections	Giving injections beneath the skin and into muscle.
21. Blood transfusion	Following the correct procedures to give a transfusion of blood into the vein of a patient (including correct identification of the patient and checking blood groups). Observation for possible reactions to the transfusion, and actions if they occur.

Therapeutic procedures (continued)

Procedure	Description in lay terms
22. Male and female urinary catheterisation	Passing a tube into the urinary bladder to permit drainage of urine, in male and female patients.
23. Instructing patients in the use of devices for inhaled medication	Providing instructions for patients about how to use inhalers correctly, for example, to treat asthma.
24. Use of local anaesthetics	Using drugs which produce numbness and prevent pain, either applied directly to the skin or injected into skin or body tissues.
25. Skin suturing	Repairing defects in the skin by inserting stitches (normally includes use of local anaesthetic).
26. Wound care and basic wound dressing	Providing basic care of surgical or traumatic wounds and applying dressings appropriately.
27. Correct techniques for 'moving and handling', including patients	Using, or directing other team members to use, approved methods for moving, lifting and handling people or objects, in the context of clinical care, using methods that avoid injury to patients, colleagues, or oneself.

General aspects of practical procedures

Aspect	Description in lay terms
28. Giving information about the procedure, obtaining and recording consent, and ensuring appropriate aftercare	Making sure that the patient is fully informed, agrees to the procedure being performed, and is cared for and watched appropriately after the procedure.
29. Hand washing (including surgical'scrubbing up')	Following approved processes for cleaning hands before procedures or surgical operations.
30. Use of personal protective equipment (gloves, gowns, masks)	Making correct use of equipment designed to prevent the spread of body fluids or cross-infection between the operator and the patient.
31. Infection control in relation to procedures	Taking all steps necessary to prevent the spread of infection before, during or after a procedure.
32. Safe disposal of clinical waste, needles and other 'sharps'	Ensuring that these materials are handled carefully and placed in a suitable container for disposal.

Appendix 2 – What the law says about undergraduate education

UK law

1   The powers and duties of the GMC in regulating medical education are set out in the Medical Act 1983.

2   From the introduction of the licence to practise, graduates who hold a UK primary medical qualification (PMQ) are entitled to provisional registration with a licence to practise, subject to demonstrating to the GMC that their fitness to practise is not impaired.

3   Standards for the delivery of the Foundation Programme, and outcomes for the training of provisionally registered doctors seeking full registration, are published under the title *The New Doctor*.

3. See GMC, *The New Doctor*

4   UK PMQs include degrees of Bachelor of Medicine and Bachelor of Surgery awarded by bodies or combinations of bodies recognised by the GMC. These are the organisations or combinations that may hold qualifying examinations. (Also, valid UK PMQs may be held by individuals who were awarded these qualifications by bodies that were at the time, but are no longer, empowered to award PMQs.)

European Union law

5   European Directive 2005/36/EC allows European Union (EU) nationals who hold an EU PMQ or specialist qualification to practise as doctors anywhere in the EU.

6   Article 24 of the Directive says the period of basic medical training must be at least six years of study or 5,500 hours of theoretical and practical training provided by, or under the supervision of, a university. From the introduction of the licence to practise, 'basic medical training' is the period leading up to full registration with a licence to practise.

7   The EU Directive says basic medical training must provide assurance that individuals acquire the following knowledge and skills:

'Adequate knowledge of the sciences on which medicine is based and a good understanding of the scientific methods including the principles of measuring biological functions, the evaluation of scientifically established facts and the analysis of data.'

'Sufficient understanding of the structure, functions and behaviour of healthy and sick persons, as well as relations between the state of health and physical and social surroundings of the human being.'

'Adequate knowledge of clinical disciplines and practices, providing him with a coherent picture of mental and physical diseases, of medicine from the points of view of prophylaxis, diagnosis and therapy and of human reproduction.'

'Suitable clinical experience in hospitals under appropriate supervision.'

These quotes have been taken from EU Directive 2005/36, Article 24.

Appendix 3 – Related documents

Undergraduate medical education: Outcomes

1   Academy of Medical Royal Colleges Intercollegiate Group on Nutrition. *Proposed Learning Objectives for the Undergraduate Medicine Nutrition Curriculum.* 2008. **www.icgnutrition.org.uk**

2   The Education Committee of the Anatomical Society of Great Britain and Ireland. 'A core syllabus in anatomy for medical students – Adding common sense to need to know.' *European Journal of Anatomy.* 2007; 11 (Supplement 1): 3-18. **www.anatsoc.org.uk**

3   Association of American Medical Colleges and Howard Hughes Medical Institute. *Scientific Foundation for Future Physicians.* 2009. **www.hhmi.org**

4   Behavioural and Social Sciences Teaching in Medicine (BeSST). *Psychology Core Curriculum for Undergraduate Medical Education.* Awaiting publication. **www.heacademy.ac.uk/besst**

5   Heads of Academic Departments of Public Health in the United Kingdom (HOADs) (original authors D Chappel, G Maudsley, R Bhopal and S Ebrahim, and re-edited by Stephen Gillam and Gillian Maudsley). *Public Health Education for Medical Students – A guide for medical schools.* Department of Public Health and Primary Care, University of Cambridge. 2008. **www.phpc.cam.ac.uk**

6   von Fragstein M., Silverman J., Cushing A., Quilligan S., Salisbury H., Wiskin C. 'UK consensus statement on the content of communication curricula in undergraduate medical education.' *Medical Education.* 2008; 42:11:1100-1107. **www3.interscience.wiley.com**

7   International Centre for Drug Policy. *Substance Misuse in the Undergraduate Medical Curriculum.* 2007. **www.sgul.ac.uk**

8   Joint Committee on Medical Genetics. *Learning Outcomes in Genetics for Medical Students.* 2006. **www.geneticseducation.nhs.uk**

9   Maxwell SRJ, Walley T. 'Teaching safe and effective prescribing in UK Medical Schools: a core curriculum for tomorrow's doctors.' *British Journal of Clinical Pharmacology.* 2003; 55:496-503. **www.bps.ac.uk**

10   Medical Schools Council. *Outcomes of the Medical Schools Council Safe Prescribing Working Group.* 2007. **www.medschools.ac.uk**

11   Royal College of Obstetricians and Gynaecologists. *National Undergraduate Curriculum in Obstetrics and Gynaecology, Report of a Working Party.* 2009. **www.rcog.org.uk**

12   Royal College of Psychiatrists. *Report of the Royal College of Psychiatrists'
Scoping Group on Undergraduate Education in Psychiatry.* 2009.
www.rcpsych.ac.uk

13   Scottish Deans' Medical Education Group. *The Scottish Doctor. Learning
Outcomes for the Medical Undergraduate in Scotland: A Foundation for
Competent and Reflective Practitioners.* 2008.
www.scottishdoctor.org

14   The Tuning Project (Medicine). *Learning Outcomes/Competences for
Undergraduate Medical Education in Europe.* Medical Education in Europe
(MEDINE), the University of Edinburgh, Education and Culture DG of the
European Commission, Tuning Educational Structures in Europe. 2008.
www.tuning-medicine.com

15   World Health Organisation World Alliance for Patient Safety. *WHO Patient
Safety Curriculum Guide for Medical Schools.* World Health Organisation.
Awaiting publication.
www.who.int

Undergraduate medical education: Delivery

16   Association for the Study of Medical Education. Series of publications on *Understanding Medical Education*. From 2006. **www.asme.org.uk**

17   Hugh Barr. *Undergraduate Interprofessional Education*. General Medical Council. 2003. **www.gmc-uk.org/education**

18   British Medical Association Medical Students Committee. *Whistle-blowing*. 2008. **www.bma.org.uk**

19   British Medical Association Medical Students Committee and Medical Schools Council. *Medical school charter*. 2006. **www.bma.org.uk**

20   Department of Health (England) and UK Centre for the Advancement of Interprofessional Education. *Creating an Interprofessional Workforce: An Education and Training Framework for Health and Social Care in England*. 2007. **www.caipe.org.uk**

21   General Medical Council. *Guidance on UK medical education delivered outside the UK*. 2008. **www.gmc-uk.org/education**

22   General Medical Council and others. *Gateways to the Professions. Advising medical schools: encouraging disabled students*. 2008. **www.gmc-uk.org/education**

23   General Medical Council and Medical Schools Council. *Medical Students: Professional Values and Fitness to Practise.* 2009.
www.gmc-uk.org/education

24   Christine Hogg. *Patient-Centred Care: Tomorrow's Doctors.* General Medical Council. 2004. **www.gmc-uk.org/education**

25   Jan Illing and others. *How prepared are medical graduates to begin practice?* General Medical Council. 2008. **www.gmc-uk.org**

26   Medical Schools Council. *Guiding Principles for the Admission of Medical Students.* 2006. **www.medschools.ac.uk**

27   Medical Schools Council. *Recommendations on Selection of Students with Specific Learning Disabilities, including Dyslexia.* 2005. **www.medschools.ac.uk**

28   Medical Schools Council. *The Ten Key Principles for joint working between the Universities and the NHS.* 2004. **www.medschools.ac.uk**

29   Medical Schools Council, the Council of Heads and Deans of Dental Schools, the Association of UK University Hospitals and the Higher Education Occupational Physicians Group. *Medical and Dental Students: Health clearance for Hepatitis B, Hepatitis C, HIV and Tuberculosis.* 2008. **www.medschools.ac.uk**

30   Anne Tynan. *Today's Disabled Students: Tomorrow's Doctors.* General
Medical Council. 2006. **www.gmc-uk.org/education**

31   World Federation for Medical Education. *Basic Medical Education:
WFME Global Standards for Quality Improvement.* 2003.
www2.sund.ku.dk/wfme

Postgraduate medical training

32   Academy of Medical Royal Colleges and the UK health departments.
The Foundation Programme Curriculum. 2007.
www.foundationprogramme.nhs.uk

33   General Medical Council. *The New Doctor.* 2007.
www.gmc-uk.org/education

34   Postgraduate Medical Education and Training Board. *Educating Tomorrow's
Doctors – Future models of medical training; medical workforce shape and
trainee expectations.* 2008.
www.pmetb.org.uk

35   Postgraduate Medical Education and Training Board. *Generic standards
for training.* 2008. **www.pmetb.org.uk**

36   Postgraduate Medical Education and Training Board. *Patients' Role in
Healthcare – The future relationship between patient and doctor.* 2008.
www.pmetb.org.uk

Medical education and training: all stages

37 Academy of Medical Royal Colleges. *Health Inequalities Curriculum Competency Project.* 2009. **www.aomrc.org.uk**

38 British Medical Association. *Equality and diversity education.* 2008. **www.bma.org.uk**

39 British Medical Association Board of Medical Education. *Doctors as teachers.* 2006. **www.bma.org.uk**

40 British Medical Association Medical Education Subcommittee. *Role of the patient in medical education.* 2008. **www.bma.org.uk**

41 Andreas Hasman, Angela Coulter, Janet Askham. *Education for Partnership. Developments in medical education.* Picker Institute Europe. 2006. **www.pickereurope.org**

42 NHS Institute for Innovation and Improvement and the Academy of Medical Royal Colleges. *Medical Leadership Competency Framework.* 2008. **www.institute.nhs.uk**

Medical practice

43   Academy of Medical Royal Colleges. *A Clinician's Guide to Record Standards.* 2008. **www.rcplondon.ac.uk**

44   British Medical Association Equal Opportunities Committee. *Career barriers in medicine.* 2004. **www.bma.org.uk**

45   British Medical Association Equal Opportunities Committee. *Disability equality in the medical profession.* 2007. **www.bma.org.uk**

46   British Medical Association Equal Opportunities Committee and Patient Liaison Group. *Disability equality within healthcare: the role of healthcare professionals.* 2007. **www.bma.org.uk**

47   General Medical Council. *Confidentiality: Protecting and providing information.* 2004. **www.gmc-uk.org/guidance**

48   General Medical Council. *Consent: Patients and doctors making decisions together.* 2008. **www.gmc-uk.org/guidance**

49   General Medical Council. *Good Medical Practice.* 2006. **www.gmc-uk.org/guidance**

50   General Medical Council. *Good practice in prescribing medicines.* 2008. **www.gmc-uk.org/guidance**

51   General Medical Council. *Personal beliefs and medical practice.* 2008. **www.gmc-uk.org/guidance**

52   General Medical Council. *Raising concerns about patient safety.* 2006.
www.gmc-uk.org/guidance

53   General Medical Council. *Research: The role and responsibilities of doctors.*
2002. **www.gmc-uk.org/guidance**

54   General Medical Council. *Withholding and withdrawing life-prolonging
treatments.* 2002. **www.gmc-uk.org/guidance**

55   Ros Levenson, Steve Dewar, Susan Shepherd. *Understanding Doctors:
Harnessing Professionalism.* King's Fund and Royal College of Physicians.
2008. **www.kingsfund.org.uk**

56   Medical Schools Council. *The Consensus Statement on the Role of the Doctor.*
2008. **www.medschools.ac.uk**

57   NHS Institute for Innovation and Improvement. *Improvement Leaders'
Guides.* 2007. **www.institute.nhs.uk**

58   Royal College of Physicians. *Doctors in society. Medical professionalism in a
changing world.* 2005. **www.rcplondon.ac.uk**

59   Royal College of Physicians. *Palliative Care Services: meeting the needs of
patients.* 2007. **www.rcplondon.ac.uk**

Higher education

60   Quality Assurance Agency. *Code of practice for the assurance of academic
quality and standards in higher education.* Various dates for sections.
www.qaa.ac.uk

Appendix 4 – Glossary

Appraisal	A positive process to provide feedback on the performance of a student or a member of staff to chart their continuing progress, and to identify their development needs.
Assessment	All activity aimed at judging students' attainment of curriculum outcomes, whether for summative purposes (determining progress) or formative purposes (giving feedback). An 'examination' is an individual assessment test.
Clinical tutor or clinical supervisor	Any doctor or other healthcare professional responsible for the supervision or assessment of a student on a placement.
Curriculum	A detailed schedule of the teaching and learning opportunities that will be provided.
Elective	A period of clinical experience that is chosen by the student and is often taken outside the UK.
Examiners	All those responsible for marking, assessing or judging students' performance, regardless of the terminology used in any particular medical school.
Integrated teaching	A system where the clinical and basic sciences are taught and learned together. This allows students to see how scientific knowledge and clinical experience are combined to support good medical practice.

Other education providers	Organisations involved in the delivery of undergraduate medical education outside the medical school itself, including their staff, GP tutors, clinical tutors, NHS staff, and others in the local health economy or independent sector with specific roles in educational supervision.
Placement	A structured period of supervised clinical experience and learning in a health or social care setting (including community health services and non-NHS settings).
Primary medical qualification (PMQ)	A first medical degree awarded by a body or combination of bodies that is recognised by the GMC for this purpose, or that was empowered to issue PMQs at the time the degree was awarded.
Revalidation	The regular demonstration by doctors that they are up to date, and fit to practise medicine.
Scheme of assessment	The examinations and assessments that make sure all students have successfully achieved and demonstrated the knowledge, skills and behaviour set out in the curriculum.
Self-directed learning	A process in which students are responsible for organising and managing their own learning activities and needs.
Student Assistantship	A period during which a student acts as assistant to a junior doctor, with defined duties under appropriate supervision.

Student-selected components (SSCs)	Parts of the curriculum that allow students to choose what they want to study. These components may also offer flexibility concerning how, where and when study will take place.

Endnotes

1   See *High Quality Care for All – NHS Next Stage Review Final Report.*

2   The term 'other education providers' means organisations involved in the delivery of undergraduate medical education outside the medical school itself, including their staff, GP tutors, clinical tutors, NHS staff, and others in the local health economy or independent sector with specific roles in educational supervision.

3   'NHS organisations' includes acute, primary care and mental health organisations, and the boards and authorities which oversee their work.

4   Primary prevention of disease is understood to refer to the prevention of disease onset. Secondary prevention of disease is understood to refer to the detection of disease in symptom-free individuals. Tertiary prevention of disease is understood to refer to the prevention of disease progression, and to palliation or rehabilitation.

5   The term 'placement' means a structured period of supervised clinical experience and learning in a health or social care setting (including community health services and non-NHS settings).

6   The terms 'clinical tutor' and 'clinical supervisor' mean any doctor or other healthcare professional responsible for the supervision or assessment of a student on a placement.

7   This includes universities and non-university bodies with appropriate degree-awarding powers that are recognised by the GMC.

8   A Student Assistantship means a period during which a student acts as assistant to a junior doctor, with defined duties under appropriate supervision.

9   A generalisable assessment is one where candidates' scores are not influenced by specific circumstances such as variability in examination conditions or examiners.

10 When acting as a Student Assistant, a student must not carry out any procedure or take responsibility for anything which requires provisional registration and, from the introduction of the licence to practise, a licence.

11 'Examiners' here means all those responsible for marking, assessing or judging students' performance, regardless of the terminology used in any particular medical school.

Index

Note: Numbers refer to page numbers